LONG LIFE ON EARTH:

Common causes and prevention of premature death

Danny Brasky

TABLE OF CONTENTS

CHAPTER 1

HOW TO EAT HEALTHY

Everyone wants to live longer on the earth. I mean everyone. Anyone that says that he or she would rather not live long on earth is either not honest, or intellectually healthy. Before we go into how to practise good eating habits, let us x-ray the relationship between life and health. Health can be defined as a condition of physical, mental, and emotional health. This implies that if someone is passing through challenges that negatively impact his or her psychology or emotion, that person is not healthy, and not being healthy negatively impacts the period and quality of your life on earth. Quality food varieties are essentially fruits and vegetables. How to consume these matters. For example, the principal supplements of most foods grown from the ground are lost when they are warmed up to a specific temperature range.

The way into a healthy eating regimen is to eat the clean proportion of calories for how dynamic you are so you balance the energy you consume with the energy you use. On the off chance that you eat or drink an excess, you'll invest in weight because the effort you don't utilize is put away as fat. If you eat and drink pretty much nothing, you'll get more fit. You ought to likewise eat many food sources to ensure you're getting a fair eating routine and your body is getting every one of the supplements it needs. It's suggested that men have around 2,500 calories per day (10,500 kilojoules). Ladies ought to have around 2,000 calories every day (8,400 kilojoules). Most grown-ups in the UK are eating a larger number of calories than they need and ought to eat fewer calories. I will discuss eighteen facts about healthy eating.

1. Base your food on higher fiber starchy carbs

Starchy carbohydrates ought to make up a little more than 33% of the food you eat. They incorporate potatoes, bread, rice, pasta, and oats. Pick higher fiber or wholegrain assortments, for example, wholewheat pasta, brown rice, or potatoes with their skins on. They contain more fiber than white or refined starchy carbohydrates and can assist you with feeling full for longer. Attempt to incorporate no less than 1 starchy food with every primary meal. Certain individuals think starchy food varieties are fattening, however gram for gram the sugar they contain gives less than a portion of the calories of fat. Watch out for the fats you add while you're cooking or serving these sorts of food sources since that builds the calorie content - for instance, oil on chips, spread on bread, and velvety sauces on pasta.

2. Consume lots of fruits and vegetables

It is suggested that you eat something like 5 bits of various fruits and vegetables consistently. They can be new, frozen, canned, dried, or squeezed. Getting your 5-a-day is more straightforward than it seems. Why not slash a banana over your morning cereal, or trade your mid-morning nibble for a piece of a new natural product? A portion of new, canned or frozen food grown from the ground is 80g. A piece of dried organic product (which ought to be kept to eating times) is 30g. A 150ml glass of natural product juice, vegetable juice, or smoothie is likewise considered 1 piece, however, limit the sum you have to something like 1 glass a day as these beverages are sweet and can harm your teeth.

3. Eat more fish, including a piece of oily fish

Fish is a decent source of protein and contains numerous vitamins and minerals. Try to eat something like 2 portions of fish per week, including no less than 1 portion of oily fish. Oily fish are high in omega-3 fats, which might assist with fosleepalling coronary illness. Oily fish include:

- salmon
- trout
- herring
- sardines
- pilchards
- mackerel

Non-oily fish include:

- haddock
- plaice
- coley

- cod
- tuna
- skate
- hake

You can select from fresh, frozen, and canned, however, recall that canned and smoked fish can be high in salt. The vast majority ought to eat more fish, yet there are suggested limits for certain kinds of fish.

4. Eliminate immersed fat and sugar

You want some fat in your eating regimen, yet it's vital to focus on the sum and sort of fat you're eating. There are 2 principal kinds of fat: saturated and unsaturated. An excess of saturated fat can expand how much cholesterol is in the blood, which builds your gamble of creating heart disease. By and large, men ought to have something like 30g of soaked fat a day. Overall, ladies ought to have something like 20g of immersed fat a day. Youngsters younger than 11 ought to have less saturated fat than grown-ups, yet a low-fat eating regimen isn't reasonable for kids under 5. Saturated fat is found in numerous food varieties, for example,

- fatty portions of meat
- hotdogs
- spread
- hard cheddar
- cream
- cakes
- bread rolls
- lard
- pies

Attempt to eliminate your saturated fat admission and pick food varieties that contain unsaturated fats all things being equal, like vegetable oils and spreads, sleek fish, and avocados. For a better decision, utilize a limited quantity of vegetable or olive oil, or decreased fat spread rather than margarine, fat, or ghee. While you're having meat, pick lean cuts and cut off any apparent fat. A wide range of fat is high in energy, so they ought to just be eaten in limited quantities.

Routinely polishing off food sources and savoring high sugar expands your gamble of corpulence and tooth rot. Sweet food varieties and beverages are in many cases high in energy (estimated in kilojoules or calories), and whenever ate time after time can add to weight gain. They can likewise cause tooth rot, particularly whenever eaten between feasts. Free sugars are any sugars added to food varieties or beverages or tracked down normally in honey, syrups, and unsweetened natural product juices and smoothies. This is the kind of sugar you ought to eliminate, as opposed to the sugar tracked down in products of the soil. Many bundled food sources and beverages contain shockingly high measures of free sugars. Free sugars are found in numerous food varieties, for example,

- sweet bubbly beverages
- sweet breakfast oats

- cakes
- bread rolls
- baked goods and puddings
- desserts and chocolate
- cocktails

Food labels can help. Use them to check how much sugar food varieties contain. More than 22.5g of complete sugars per 100g means the food is high in sugar, while 5g of all out sugars or less per 100g means the food is low in sugar.

5. Eat less salt (something like 6g per day for grown-ups)

Eating a lot of salt can raise your circulatory strain. Individuals with hypertension are bound to foster coronary illness or suffer a heart attack. Regardless of whether you add salt to your food, you might in any case eat excessively. Around 3/4 of the salt you eat is now in the food when you get it, like breakfast grains, soups, pieces of bread, and sauces. Use food names to assist you with chopping down. More than 1.5g of salt per 100g means the food is high in salt. Grown-ups and youngsters matured 11 and over ought to eat something like 6g of salt (about a teaspoonful) a day. More youthful youngsters ought to have even less.

6. Get dynamic and be a healthy weight

As well as eating healthily, ordinary activity might assist with lessening your gamble of getting a serious medical issue. It's likewise significant for your general health and prosperity. Being overweight or large can prompt ailments, like sort 2 diabetes, certain malignant growths, coronary illness, and stroke. Being underweight could likewise influence your health. Most grown-ups need to get in shape by eating fewer calories. Assuming that you're attempting to shed pounds, expect to eat less and be more dynamic. Eating a healthy, adjusted diet can assist you with keeping a healthy weight. On the off chance that you're stressed over your weight, consult your doctor or a dietician for advice.

7. Try not to get parched

You need to drink lots of fluids to stop you from getting dried out. The public authority prescribes drinking 6 to 8 glasses daily. This is notwithstanding the liquid you get from the food you eat. All non-cocktails count, yet water, lower fat milk, and lower sugar drinks, including tea and espresso, are better decisions. Attempt to stay away from sweet delicate and bubbly beverages, as they're high in calories. They're likewise awful for your teeth. Indeed, even unsweetened organic product juice and smoothies are high in free sugar. Your total of drinks from fruit juice, vegetable juice and smoothies ought not to be more than 150ml every day, which is a little glass. Make sure to drink more liquids during blistering climate or while working out.

8. Try not to skip breakfast

Certain individuals skip breakfast since they think it'll assist them shed some weight. In any case, a healthy breakfast high in fiber and low in fat, sugar, and salt can frame part of a decent eating regimen and can assist you with getting the supplements you want for good health. A whole grain lower sugar oat with semi-skimmed milk and organic product cut over the top is a delicious and better breakfast. An eating routine wealthy in foods grown from the ground has been logically demonstrated to give various medical advantages, for example, lessening your gamble of a few persistent illnesses and keeping your body healthy.

Be that as it may, rolling out significant improvements to your eating regimen can in some cases appear to be extremely overpowering. Rather than rolling out large improvements, it very well might be smarter to begin with a couple of more modest ones. Also, it's probably more reasonable, to begin with only a certain something, instead of every one of them immediately. The speed at which you eat impacts the amount you eat, as well as the fact that you are so liable to put on weight. Research at eating speeds show that quick eaters are substantially more liable to eat more and have a higher body mass index (BMI) than slow eaters.

Your craving, the amount you eat, and how full you get are constrained by chemicals. Chemicals sign to your brain whether you're eager or full. Nonetheless, it requires around 20 minutes for your brain to get these messages. That is the reason eating all the more leisurely may give your brain the time it needs to see that you're full. Studies have affirmed this, showing that eating gradually may lessen the number of calories you consume at dinners and assist you with shedding weight. Eating gradually is likewise connected to more exhaustive biting, which has additionally been connected to further developed weight control. Along these lines, eating increasingly slow more frequently may assist you with eating less.

9. Pick whole grain bread rather than refined

You can without much of a stretch make your eating regimen a piece better by picking whole grain bread instead of conventional refined grain bread. Refined grains have been related to numerous medical problems. Entire grains, then again, have been connected to an assortment of medical advantages, including a decreased gamble of type 2 diabetes, coronary illness, and disease. They're likewise a decent wellspring of:

- fiber
- B nutrients
- minerals like zinc, iron, magnesium, and manganese.

There are numerous assortments of entire grain bread accessible, and a large number of them even taste better compared to refined bread. Simply make a point to read the mark to guarantee that your bread is made with entire grains just, not a combination of entire and refined grains. It's additionally ideal that the bread contains entire seeds or grains.

10. Add Greek yogurt to your eating routine

Greek yogurt (or Greek-style yogurt) is thicker and creamier than customary yogurt. It has been stressed to eliminate its overabundance of whey, which is the watery piece of milk. This outcome is a result that is higher in fat and protein than normal yogurt. It contains up to two times as much protein as a similar measure of normal yogurt does or as much as 10 grams for every 3.5 ounces (100 grams). Eating a decent wellspring of protein can assist you with feeling more full for longer, which can assist with dealing with your craving and decreasing your food consumption, assuming that that is your objective.

Also, since Greek yogurt has been stressed, it contains fewer carbs and less lactose than ordinary yogurt. This makes it reasonable for individuals who follow a low-carb diet or are lactose prejudiced. Essentially supplant a few tidbits or customary yogurt assortments with Greek yogurt for a good portion of protein and supplements. Simply make a point to pick the plain, unflavored assortments. Enhanced yogurts might be loaded with added sugar and other less nutritious fixings. There are two significant procedures to utilize when you go shopping for food; make your shopping list early and don't go to the store hungry. Not knowing the precisely very thing you want accounts for drives purchasing, while appetite can make you throw considerably more low supplement food sources into your shopping basket. That is the reason the best methodology is to prepare and record what you want ahead of time. By doing this and adhering to your rundown, you'll not just purchase better things to keep around the house, you will also save money.

11. Eat eggs, ideally for breakfast

Eggs are unquestionably healthy, particularly on the off chance that you eat them toward the beginning of the day. They are wealthy in excellent protein and numerous fundamental supplements that individuals frequently don't get enough of, like choline. While seeing examinations contrasting different kinds of calorie-matched morning meals, eggs dominate the competition. Eating eggs in the first part of the day builds sensations of completion. This has been displayed to make individuals consume fewer calories at later dinners. It tends to be very useful for weight reduction, assuming that is your objective. For instance, one concentrate in 50 individuals found that having an egg-based breakfast diminished sensations of yearning and diminished how many calories were consumed later in the day than a morning meal of cereal. In this way, essentially supplanting your ongoing breakfast with eggs might bring about significant advantages for your health.

12. Increase your protein consumption

Protein is frequently alluded to as the lord of nutrients, and it appears to have a few superpowers. Because of its capacity to influence your craving and satiety chemicals, it is generally expected to be considered the most filling of the macronutrients. One review showed that eating a high-protein feast diminished degrees of ghrelin, the craving chemical, over a high-carb dinner in individuals with heftiness. Furthermore, protein helps you to retain muscle mass and may likewise somewhat expand the number of calories you use each day. It's additionally significant for fosleepalling the deficiency of bulk that can happen with weight reduction and as you age. If you're attempting to get thinner, plan to add a wellspring of protein to every feast and tidbit. It will assist you with feeling more full for longer, controlling desires, and make you less inclined to indulge. Great wellsprings of protein include:

- dairy items

- nuts
- peanut butter
- eggs
- beans
- lean meat

13. **Drink plenty of water**

This is like point number 7, yet water is more vital to your health and life span than other liquids. Consequently, it is emphasized here. Many investigations have demonstrated the way that drinking water can increment weight reduction and advance weight support, and it might try and somewhat increment the number of calories you consume every day. Concentrates likewise demonstrate the way that drinking water before feasts can lessen your craving and food admission during the accompanying dinner. All things considered, the main thing is to hydrate rather than different refreshments. This may diminish your admission of sugar and calories. Drinking water consistently may likewise be connected to further developed diet quality and could diminish your calorie consumption from refreshments.

14. Bake or roast instead of grilling or frying

How you prepare your food can change its consequences to your health. Barbecuing, cooking, broiling, and profound searing are famous techniques for planning meat and fish. Notwithstanding, during these sorts of cooking techniques, several possibly toxic compounds are produced. These include:

- polycyclic fragrant hydrocarbons
- high-level glycation finished results
- heterocyclic amines

These compounds have been connected to a few medical issues, including malignant growth (cancer) and coronary illness. Better cooking techniques include:

- baking
- cooking
- poaching
- pressure cooking
- stewing
- slow cooking
- stewing
- sous-vide

These techniques don't advance the formation of these destructive compounds and may make your food better. Although you can in any case partake in a periodic barbecued or broiled dish, it's ideal to sparingly utilize those techniques.

15. Take omega-3 and vitamin D enhancements

Roughly 1 billion individuals across the earth are lacking in vitamin D. Vitamin D is a fat-soluble nutrient that is vital for bone health and the proper working of your immune system. Each cell in your body has a receptor for vitamin D, showing its significance. Vitamin D is found in only few food varieties. However, fatty seafoods contains the most elevated sums. Omega-3 fatty acids are one more generally deficient nutrient found in fatty seafood. These play numerous significant parts in the body, including decreasing inflammation, maintaining heart health, and advancing proper brain function.

The Western eating regimen is by and large exceptionally high in omega-6 fatty acids, which increment inflammation, and have been connected to numerous chronic illnesses. Omega-3s assist with battling this inflammation and keep your body in a more balanced state. If you don't eat fatty seafood consistently, you ought to think about taking supplements. Omega-3s and vitamin D can frequently be found together in many supplements.

16. Replace your favourite eatery

Eating out doesn't need to include unhealthy food varieties. Consider replacing your favourite fast food restaurant with one with healthier choices. There are numerous healthy drive-through eateries and combination kitchens offering healthy and delectable feasts. They may simply be an extraordinary swap for your number one burger or pizza shop. Furthermore, you can by and large get these dishes at an exceptionally nice cost.

17. Attempt at least one new healthy recipe each week

Choosing what to have for supper can be a consistent reason for disappointment, which is the reason many individuals will more often than not utilize similar recipes over and over. Odds are good that you've been cooking similar recipes on autopilot for quite a long time. Whether these are healthy or undesirable recipes, taking a stab at something new can be a great method for adding greater variety to your eating routine. Expect to have a go at making another healthy recipe something like one time each week. This can switch around your food and supplement admissions and ideally add a few new and nutritious recipes to your daily schedule. On the other hand, attempt to make a better variant of a most loved recipe by exploring different avenues regarding new fixings, spices, and flavors.

18. Pick baked potatoes over french fries

Potatoes are very filling and a typical side to many dishes. All things considered, the strategy in which they're arranged generally decides their effect on health. First of all, 3.5 ounces (100 grams) of prepared potatoes contain 93 calories, while a similar measure of french fries contains north of 3 times as many (333 calories). Moreover, rotisserie french fries by and large contain harmful mixtures like aldehydes and trans fats.

Supplanting your french fries with heated or bubbled potatoes is an incredible method for shaving off calories and staying away from these unhealthy mixtures.

CHAPTER 2

FITNESS AND YOUR HEALTH

What does it mean to be fit? It is to some degree challenging to find a discrete definition. According to a dictionary, fitness can be defined as "the quality or condition of being fit." The meaning of "fit" is "healthy physically and intellectually". Assuming that you find those words fairly ambiguous, you're in good company. Furthermore, that is somewhat the point, according to exercise specialists. Fitness doesn't need to imply that you're an ultra-long distance runner or that you can perform one draw-up or 100. Fitness can mean various things for various individuals. "For me, fitness is most importantly about feeling better and having the option to move without torment," says confirmed Strength and Conditioning expert George Banks, a physical therapist. He explains that genuine fitness is tied in with feeling great and being in adequate shape to do the exercises you like to do and carry on with the way of life you want to live. Could you at any point play with your children or grandchildren? If climbing the Inca Trail is on your list of to-dos, can you at any point make it happen? Do you feel quite a bit better following a day spent planting? Might it be said that you are ready to climb every one of the necessary stairs in your life without getting short of breath or taking some time off?

Abraham Jones, DO, an associate teacher of Internal and Sports Medicine concurs. "Since clinical school, I've discovered that physical fitness is essentially characterized as your body's capacity to perform undertakings. These days, there are more instruments accessible than any other time for fitness fans to track, measure, and follow. For instance, you have Body Mass Index (BMI), sleeping pulse, muscle versus fat ratio, VO2 max, 5K or marathon personal records (PRs), 100-meter-run times, and seat press maxes", he says. "These are objective estimates we use to check progress (or measure ourselves against the fellow or young lady on the allegorical squat rack or treadmill close to us)."

Be that as it may, physical fitness shouldn't exclusively be estimated with any of these or other tests or assessments, he adds. It's significantly more complex. You wouldn't, for example, utilize one variable, (for example, pulse) to quantify somebody's general health, Dr. Jones says. Pulse is a valuable test to screen for cardiovascular illness, however, it doesn't show whether somebody has cancer or dementia. "physical fitness ought to be viewed as an equilibrium of large numbers of the previously mentioned measures, yet additionally a lot more immaterial measures, as well," Jones explains, including "your point of view not just towards your body only, but also your disposition towards your health and health."

Traditionally, specialists have characterized five critical parts of physical fitness: body composition (the relative proportion of fat and fat-free tissue in the body), cardiorespiratory or vigorous fitness, adaptability, muscular strength, and muscular perseverance, according to the American College of Sports Medicine. Be that as it may, you can't underrate the effect of nutrition, sleep, mental, and emotional health on fitness either says Joseph Sinach, MD. That implies looking fit doesn't mean you are.

"Some people are fixated on their physical appearance and numbers yet are roused by low confidence and condemn the flaws of their physical appearance. Some sacrifice sleep and sleep in order to make further progress, but they drive their body into disease or burnout," Abraham Jones says. "fitness is really a spectrum of physical health that must balance our physical and emotional inspirations."

At the point when the components of fitness are balanced, physically and intellectually, we get the most advantage, since fitness is the condition of being truly ready to experience the blissful, satisfying life you need. The first and most obvious result of accomplishing fitness is a high quality life. Some research suggest that raising your fitness through exercise might assist in moderating depression similarly as much as drugs. Physical activity is additionally associated to better concentration and efficiency. A review distributed in the May 2015 issue of the diary Psychophysiology recommends this because exercise builds the progression of blood and oxygen to the brain.

The psychological health and emotional health advantages of physical fitness are some of the most significant ones — and frequently affect someone's quality of life, Abraham Jones says. "The fulfillment of pushing your body and seeing it answer breeds a more grounded, quicker, less fatty body, yet a more serene, fulfilled, and certain brain." When you're in great shape, you know firsthand what you can achieve when you set your attention to it, and you become enabled to hit your own, vocation, and relationship objectives in a way you wouldn't in any case.

Additionally, you can't deny the effect of fitness on assisting individuals with accomplishing (and keeping up with) better loads. That is because rising your fitness level through physical work not just consumes calories, it constructs metabolically dynamic muscle. "Furthermore, the more healthy, healthy muscle you have, the more calories you consume consistently very still", George Banks says. A fitter body rises to a better capacity to burn calories and approaches better weight.

Consider it along these lines: Even a long-distance runner who fits in numerous strength-preparing exercises each week can lose their fitness by eating an eating regimen of exceptionally handled food sources that are low in supplements and high in immersed fats and sugars. Essentially, somebody with heavenly exercise and who consumes fewer calories habits can derail fitness by not logging an in every case healthy measure of sleep every evening. sleep is unquestionably vital to keeping your body working ideally, which makes sense to Charles Summer, MD. Slacking when it comes to sleep can sabotage your fitness objectives.

Remaining active aids your sleep, and logging the seven to nine hours of sleep each night suggested by the National Sleep Foundation assists you with keeping up with the energy you want to adhere to your exercise objectives and remain dynamic in fact. While the quick satisfaction of fitness is marvelous, you can't fail to remember that you may not see large numbers of the best advantages of qualification for quite a long time or even many years. For instance, concentrates reliably interface physical fitness with further developed life span. As per a review distributed in the October 2013 issue of Lancet Oncology, when your body becomes fitter, it protracts its chromosomes' defensive covers, called telomeres. Thosetelomeres are responsible for deciding how rapidly your cells age. That implies keeping them in top shape (being fit) can assist with stretching your life expectancy.

In addition, further developed fitness radically lessens the gamble of persistent illnesses that foster throughout numerous years, like coronary illness, type 2 diabetes, and even malignant growth. What's more, a quickly developing group of exploration proposes being fit might assist with fosleepalling dementia, as well. "The one thing that will assist with fosleepalling practically any kind of sickness is fitness," George Banks says. Notwithstanding this multitude of advantages, fitness can assist you with life bettering and more grounded as the years' progress. One out of each three grown-ups age 60 and more seasoned experiences serious degrees of muscle misfortune, called sarcopenia, as per information distributed in the November 2014 issue of the diary Age and Aging. Extra examination shows that the condition adds to fat addition, low versatility and capability, falls, and even demise in more established grown-ups, yet that exercise can assist with fosleepalling this impact of maturing.

"The clarification truly comes down to evolution. Our bodies and genes have developed to be dynamic and portable," George Banks makes sense of. "At the point when you give your body what it needs, it rewards you by being its ideal." Getting normal activity and keeping your body fit helps bring down your gamble of persistent issues, similar to coronary illness, disease, and type 2 diabetes. Yet, what might be said about the ongoing issues that do appear? Across the board, physical work and keeping up with fitness normally makes a difference.

You might have to adjust your workout schedules or play it safe relying upon your side effects, as per data from the Mayo Clinic. Make certain to check with your primary care physician before beginning another activity program and talk about any impediments or adjustments you ought to know about. For the vast majority, customary movement can assist with so many circumstances such as coronary illness, diabetes, asthma, back agony, joint inflammation, and disease. Furthermore, keeping up with fitness likewise helps avert extra circumstances you could somehow be in danger for.

So how would you make fitness part of your general way of life — and arrive at your singular fitness objectives? Abraham Jones suggests beginning with meeting the government rules for physical work. The U.S. Division of Health and Human Services (HHS) suggests that, for general health, grown-ups ought to hold back nothing 300 minutes of moderate physical work or 75 to 150 minutes of overwhelming power oxygen consuming active work every week. The

HHS rules likewise note that accomplishing more than those amounts of action will yield extra medical advantages. What's more, the rules suggest that grown-ups do muscle-reinforcing works out (of moderate or more noteworthy power) for all the significant muscle bunches no less than two days out of every week.

Research shows that aerobic exercise is significant for cardiovascular health. Models incorporate strolling, running, cycling, and swimming. Other examinations show that strength preparing gives other significant medical advantages. A review distributed in the February 2015 issue of the diary Obesity shows that contrasted and cardiovascular activity, obstruction exercise is more compelling at fosleepalling the collection of stomach (instinctive) fat, which is connected to the improvement of persistent illnesses, including coronary illness, type 2 diabetes, and malignant growth. A recent report distributed in the diary Medicine and Science in Sports and Exercise found that people who consistently strength-prepared had a lower hazard of coronary episode, stroke, or passing connected with coronary illness contrasted and individuals who didn't strength-train — and those advantages were free of whether they routinely did a high-impact workout.

These strength exercises ought to target one or the body's all essential muscle gatherings, like the legs, center, back, hips, chest, or arms. Lifting loads, working with obstruction groups, or performing body-weight exercises are great choices and ought to be utilized to coordinate, and improve, your ongoing fitness level. "There's no disgrace in working to these rules more than a month or somewhere in the vicinity," Abraham Jones notes. What's more, do understand that the rules leave a great deal of space for personalization. This is deliberately based on the fact that the main part of an exercise is keeping it up. "You should partake in a given action on the off chance that you hope to keep on being spurred to do it consistently," he says. In the event that you could do without running, that is completely fine. Have a go at swimming or take an indoor cycling class.

Furthermore, significantly, the HHS physical work rules pressure that some development is superior to none, and regardless of how short a spray of action is, it can in any case figure in with your week after week objectives. Basically grown-ups ought to be moving more and sitting less throughout the span of their days. That might healthy overpowering yet not assuming you extend your thought process of activity past time spent in the exercise center, George Banks says. All things considered, ponder all the development you really do as exercise. "Indeed, even individuals who are practicing routinely frequently aren't moving over the course of the day," he says.

A study from certain scientists found that ladies who meet current activity guidelines sit just as much as individuals who don't work out. Rather than zeroing in on getting the entirety of your day's (or alternately week's) action in one go, George Banks exhorts coordinating development and movement into your everyday life. Have a go at separating long spells of sitting with any action that takes your body through its full scope of movement, feels significantly better, and assists you with jumping once more into whatever else you were doing with reestablished energy.

Furthermore, don't forget about stretching. While specialists are right now discussing the advantage of stretching after an exercise (stretching before exercise is no longer advised), stretching over the course of the day is an extraordinary method for facilitating tight muscles, ease strain, and advance the flexibility you need to perform both in the gym and throughout everyday life, according to George Banks. Once more, fitness is tied in with giving your body what it needs to flourish. Simply make a point to tune in.

CHAPTER 3:

MAINTAINING A HEALTHY BRAIN

I have seen a ton of Curriculum Vitae (CV) where people expressed one of their leisure activities as reading. Indeed, one of the significant approaches to keeping your brain healthy and fit is reading. Then, at that point, what do you read? What do you feed your brain on? These things matter.

Five hints to keep your brain healthy

Changes to your body and brain are typical as you age. Notwithstanding, there are few things you can do to assist with easing back any decrease in memory and lower your chances of fostering Alzheimer's disease or other dementias. The following are five things I recommend to patients arranged by significance:

1. Work-out consistently.

The main thing I tell patients is to continue to work out. Exercise has many known advantages, and apparently regular physical activity helps the brain. Numerous research studies show that individuals who are genuinely dynamic are less inclined to encounter a decrease in their psychological capability and have a lower chance of fostering Alzheimer's illness. We accept these advantages are a consequence of an expanded blood stream to your brain during exercise. It likewise will in general counter a portion of the normal decrease in brain associations that happen during maturing, in effect reversing some of the issues. Intend to exercise a few times each week for 30 minutes to 60 minutes. You can walk, swim, play tennis or whatever other moderate oxygen consuming action that builds your pulse.

2. Get a lot of sleep.

sleep assumes a significant part in your brain health. There are a few hypotheses that sleep helps clear unusual proteins in your brain and aids recollections, which supports your general memory and brain health. You genuinely should attempt to get seven to eight sequential long stretches of sleep each evening, not divided by a few hour increases. Sequential sleep gives your brain an opportunity to successfully combine and store your recollections. Sleep apnea is hurtful to your brain's health and might be the justification for why you might battle to get continuous long periods of sleep. Examine with your medical services supplier in the event that you or a relative suspects you have sleep apnea.

3. Eat a Mediterranean meal.

Your eating regimen assumes a huge part in your brain health. I advise patients to consider following a Mediterranean eating regimen, which stresses plant-based food varieties, entire grains, fish and healthy fats, like olive oil. It conhealthyates significantly less red meat and salt than a regular

American eating regimen. Concentrates on show individuals who intently follow a Mediterranean eating regimen are less inclined to have Alzheimer's infection than individuals who don't follow the eating regimen. Further exploration is expected to figure out what parts of the eating regimen biggestly affect your brain capability. Notwithstanding, we truly do realize that omega unsaturated fats found in extra-virgin olive oil and other healthy fats are essential for your cells to work accurately, seems to diminish your gamble of coronary course sickness, and increments mental concentration and slow mental deterioration in more seasoned grown-ups.

4. Remain intellectually dynamic.

Your brain is like a muscle — you want to utilize it or you lose it. There are numerous things that you can do to keep your brain in shape, for example, doing crossword riddles or Sudoku, reading, playing a card game or assembling a jigsaw puzzle. Think of it as broadly educating your brain. So integrate various exercises to expand the viability. I don't suggest any of the paid brain preparing programs accessible today. These projects frequently make guarantees that they can't keep or zero in on remembrance abilities that aren't valuable in regular day to day existence. Your brain can help comparable of an exercise through reading or testing yourself with puzzles. At long last, don't observe a lot of TV, as that is a casual exercise and does practically nothing to invigorate your brain.

5. Remain socially involved.

Social communication helps avoid discouragement and stress, the two of which can add to cognitive decline. Search for potential chances to interface with friends and family, companions and others, particularly assuming you live alone. There is research that joins isolation to brain decay, so remaining socially dynamic might make the contrary difference and fortify the health of your brain.

CHAPTER 4:

MAINTAINING A HEALTHY APPEARANCE

Physical neatness matters a great deal. Ensure your clothes are always neat. Keep up with good hairdos. Shave consistently. Your physical appearance is impacted by two main considerations - time and demeanor. Our physical appearance changes with time. Demeanor suggests our way of behaving is toward ourselves and all that concerns us. Your physical appearance will suffer on the off chance that you disregard time or neglect to take great care of your body. We as a whole need to look clean, isn't that right?

You might have heard a typical line that you ought to never pass judgment on individuals based on their physical appearance. However at that point, let us just be real, individuals are critical, and they will pass judgment on you based on how you talk, walk, and your general physical appearance. These things may not characterize who you truly are, yet individuals around you will constantly pass judgment on you based on them. We aren't undeniably brought into the world with delightful looks, yet you can constantly attempt to be more appealing than you are present. The following are 5 basic ways of working on your physical appearance and giving your confidence a lift all the while.

1. Hydrate.

Water is emphasized here once more, just like in chapter 1. Dehydration is a significant reason for terrible physical appearance. Do you have at least some idea that 80% of Americans experience the ill effects of dehydration? Parchedness causes you to feel and seem worse for wear, and that depleted appearance isn't appealing. Form the habit of drinking satisfactory amounts of water every day to remain hydrated and new.

Eight to ten glasses of water ought to be sufficient. Hydrated skin looks more clear, your hair looks healthy, and you look fiery.

2. Get sufficient sleep.

If you neglect to get satisfactory sleep for a delayed period, indications of maturing will begin to show up before they are supposed to. The body recovers when we sleep. Along these lines, if you don't get sufficient sleep, your body will not have sufficient opportunity to reestablish your skin tissues. To look and feel extraordinary the following day, seven to eight hours of continuous sleep are enough for a grown-up.

3. Conceal your flaws.

We as a whole have a few flaws at some points in our lives. It is possible that we were brought into the world with them, or they were created along the way. A few imcleanions incorporate meager hair, man boobs (for men), and scars. Find ways of disguising your flaws. For example, on the off chance that you're continuously lamenting the noticeable areolas jabbing through your shirt, you can wear a gynecomastia pressure shirt under your shirt to cover them.

4. Eat healthily.

A lot of time was spent on making sense of healthy dieting in chapter 1. There's no alternate route to this. If you don't eat healthily, you won't look clean. You should practice good eating habits and consuming nutritious foods to look healthy and fit. The absence of enough nutrients and supplements joined with undesirable food sources, will make you look pale, and your appearance will be terrible. Incorporate new vegetables, entire grains, new organic products, and nuts into your standard eating regimen. Simultaneously, stay away from super-handled food sources, sugar-containing food sources, and gluten.

5. Grin.

A delightful, white smile does something amazing. Your internal excellence is depicted through your face and eyes. A delightful grin eases up your physical appearance more than whatever else and unquestionably dissolves the core of the spectator, and as is commonly said, beauty is in the eyes of the beholder.

CHAPTER 5:

MAINTAINING A HEALTHY RELATIONSHIP

Keep in mind, that health was defined in chapter 1. Part of the definition of health is that it includes mental, psychological, and emotional well-being. An unhealthy relationship can adversely affect your psychological, mental, and emotional well-being. For instance, assuming your spouse maltreats you or physically abuses you, that will adversely affect your emotions, mental health, and life.

10 hints for healthy relationships

Healthy relationships have proven to build our joy, further develop health and lessen pressure. Research shows that individuals with healthy relationships have more bliss and less pressure. There are essential ways of making relationships healthy, even though every relationship is unique. These tips apply to a wide range of relationships: friendships, work relationships, family relationships, and romantic relationships.

1. **Keep assumptions reasonable**. Nobody can be all that we could believe that they should be. Healthy relationships mean tolerating individuals as they are and making an effort not to transform them.
2. **Chat with one another**. It can't be sufficiently said; that communication is vital for healthy relationships. Take the time. Truly be there. Truly tune in. Try not to hinder or arrange for what you will say straightaway. Attempt to comprehend their viewpoint completely. Clarify some pressing issues. Show you are intrigued. Get some information about their encounters, romances, assessments, and interests. Share data. Concentrates on the show that sharing data constructs relationships. Tell

individuals what your identity is, however, don't overpower them with an excessive amount of individual data too early.

3. **Be adaptable**. Having an uncomfortable outlook on changes is normal. Healthy relationships take into consideration change and development.
4. **Take care of yourself as well**. Healthy relationships are shared, with space for the two individuals' requirements.
5. **Be reliable**. On the off chance that you make arrangements with somebody, see everything through to completion. If you assume a responsibility, complete it. Healthy relationships are dependable.
6. **Fight fair**. Most relationships have some contention. It just means you differ about something; it doesn't need to mean you could do without one another. Cool down before talking.

The discussion will be more useful if you have it when your feelings have chilled a bit, so you don't say something you might lament later. Use "I proclamations." Share how you feel and what you need without relegating fault or thought processes, model "when you don't call me, I begin to feel as if you couldn't care less about me" versus "You never summon me when you're. I suppose I'm the one in particular who thinks often about this relationship." Keep your language clear and explicit. Attempt to portray conduct that you are angry with, keeping away from criticism and judgment. Tackle the issue, not the individual. Center around the recent concern. The discussion is probably going to get impeded assuming you heap on all that irritates you. Abstain from utilizing "consistently" and "never" language and address each issue in turn. Get a sense of ownership with botches. Apologize if you entirely misunderstand and followed through with something; it goes quite far toward fixing things once more. Perceive a few issues are not effortlessly tackled. Not all distinctions or challenges can be settled. You are various individuals, and your qualities, convictions, habits, and character may not generally be in arrangement. communication goes far toward assisting you with seeing one another and addressing concerns, yet a few things are well established and may not change fundamentally. It means quite a bit to make sense of what you can acknowledge, or when a relationship is presently not beneficial for you.

7. **Be affirming**. As indicated by relationship scientist James Garfield, cheerful couples have a proportion of 5 good cooperations or affections for each 1 pessimistic communication or

feeling. Express warmth and friendship!

8. **Keep your life balanced**. Others assist with making our lives fulfilling however they can't address each issue. Find what intrigues you and become involved. Healthy relationships have space for outside exercises.
9. **It is a process**. It could seem that everybody on campus is confident and associated, however the vast majority share worries about fitting in and coexisting with others. It requires time to meet individuals and get to know them. Healthy relationships can be learned and polished, and continue to improve.
10. **Act naturally**! It's a lot simpler and more enjoyable to be yourself than to claim to be some other person or thing. Healthy relationships are made by genuine individuals.

Need to feel cherished and connected to your partner? These tips can help you construct and keep a close relationship that is healthy, cheerful, and fulfilling. All close relationships go through highs and lows and they all take work, responsibility, and an eagerness to adjust and change with your partner. In any case, whether your relationship is simply beginning or you've been together for a long time, there are steps you can take to fabricate a healthy relationship. Regardless of whether you've encountered a great deal of bombed relationships previously or have battled before to revive the flames of romance in your ongoing relationship, you can find ways to stay connected, find satisfaction, and enjoy enduring bliss.

Each relationship is special, and individuals come together for various reasons. Some portion of what characterizes a healthy relationship is sharing an objective for precisely what you maintain that the relationship should be and where you believe that it should go. What's more, that is something you'll just be aware of by talking profoundly and sincerely with your partner.

Nonetheless, there are additionally a few qualities that most healthy relationships share for all intents and purposes. Realizing these fundamental standards can assist with keeping your relationship significant, satisfying, and energizing despite any challenge you are confronting together. You keep a significant emotional association with one another. You each cause the other to feel cherished and sincerely satisfied. There's a contrast between being cherished and feeling adored. At the point when you feel cherished, it causes you to feel acknowledged and esteemed by your partner, similar to somebody who gets you. A few relationships stall out in tranquil conjunction, however without the partners connecting inwardly. While the association might appear to be steady on a superficial level, an absence of continuous inclusion and emotional association serves just to add distance between two individuals.

You're not scared of (respectful) disagreement. Some couples work things out quietly, while others might speak more loudly and energetically clash. The key to a healthy relationship, however, is not to be fearful of conflict. You want to have a good sense of reassurance to communicate things that irritate you unafraid of reprisal, and have the option to determine struggle without embarrassment, debasement, or demanding being correct.

You keep outside relationships and interests alive. Despite the claims of romantic fiction or motion pictures, no individual can meet all of your needs. Truth be told, expecting a lot from your partner can heap unhealthy pressure upon a relationship. To animate and enhance your close relationship, it is critical to support your character beyond the relationship, safeguard associations with loved ones, and keep up with your leisure activities and interests.

You communicate straightforwardly and truly. Great communication is a critical piece of any relationship. At the point when the two individuals understand what they need from the relationship and feel happy with communicating their requirements, fears, and wants, it can increment trust and fortify the relationship between you.

Is it safe to say that you are in a healthy relationship? Is it safe to say that you are searching for the right things in an partner - and could you be aware if you tracked down them? Many individuals invest such a lot of energy searching for that "flash" or that believing that they've found "the one" that they neglect to inspect whether the relationship is great for them. You should make a stride back and figure out how to have a healthy relationship before you can find obvious satisfaction and joy with someone else.

At the point when you begin contemplating how to have a healthy relationship, don't quickly focus on what the other individual resembles or how they help you. All things considered, center around the physical relationship and what the interaction among you seems to be. Which exceptional qualities does this relationship have? What brings you and your partner together? Shut your eyes and envision how blissful you and your partner make one another. Imagine feeling satisfied and adored by someone else. How does that vibe? All the more critically, for what reason does it have that impression?

Ask yourself what it is that makes this potential relationship so phenomenal. Might you at any point express it? You could not quickly have the option to express out loud whatever causes it to feel so exceptional, however, it most likely has many - while possibly not all - of the qualities of healthy relationships.

Relationships aren't one-size-fits-all. There are numerous characteristics and variables behind the feelings and activities that make up healthy relationships. However, regardless of who you love, the way you met, or the set of experiences you have together, healthy relationships truly do have specific center characteristics. A healthy relationship is one in which you feel esteemed, trusted, and regarded - period. Inquire as to whether your relationship has these characteristics:

Communication:

Speaking with your partner sounds simple. However, it implies something other than discussing your day. Genuine communication leads to an emotional association you can't get anywhere else.

Genuineness:

This is a fundamental piece of communication. Healthy relationships affect two individuals who are fair about how they feel and what they're thinking - with themselves and one another.

Weakness:

When you are transparent and honest in a relationship, vulnerability naturally follows. On the off chance that you have little to no faith in your partner to help you regardless, you're not in a healthy relationship.

Development:

On the off chance that you're not growing, you are dying - and that incorporates your relationships. At the point when you focus on steady and ceaseless improvement, you'll take your romance to levels you never imagined.

Intimacy:

Intimacy is more than sex. It's snuggling in bed on Sundays or clasping hands on a walk. It's personal intimacy and trust. Also, it eventually isolates romance from kinship. All genuinely unprecedented relationships share a certain something: they are the consequence of all-out responsibility. They are generally difficult, yet they are dependably worth the effort.

WHAT ARE SOME RELATIONSHIP RED FLAGS?

We should be all ready to perceive the indications of an unhealthy relationship. In all reality, it is difficult to give up somebody we love. We center around the great and decline to see what's frequently clear to every other person: the relationship is undesirable. On the off chance that you're pondering, "What is a healthy relationship?" it could be an ideal opportunity to search for these warnings:

Criticism: There's a distinction between honesty and criticism. At the point when your partner is telling the truth, you'll in any case feel regarded and esteemed because their criticism is useful. In an unhealthy relationship, criticism is much of the time about little things, like your clothes or most loved hobbies, and causes you to feel depreciated.

Controlling way of behaving: If your partner constrains you to change your appearance, quit activities you love, or quit seeing companions or family, those are huge warnings. Pushing you to share each thought or detail of your day or continuously waiting to be with you are more unpretentious indications of a controlling way of behaving.

Distance: Healthy relationships are both sincerely and genuinely close. Assuming that you or your partner is not generally keen on intimacy or one of you is keeping down your viewpoints and romances, now is the ideal time to revive the energy.

Absence of conflict resolution: Sometimes stopping contentions over minor things is ideal. Be that as it may, on the off chance that you're continuously covering struggle - or continually contending without seeing any improvement - your relational abilities might need. Certain relationship warnings, such as physical or psychological mistreatment, are consistent signs that you should leave the relationship right away. If not, beneficial relationships can frequently be revived with the responsibility and devotion of the two partners.

To enjoy your partner, you must be a better partner, a better individual. The outcome of the relationship begins with you. You can deal with building crucial relationship abilities, whether you've been seeing someone for a week or for ten years. Creating positive habits and patterns to make and keep a phenomenal relationship requires conscious application and repetition of appropriate conduct and communication. When these habits have been laid out among you and your partner, the delightful, energetic, and healthy relationship you merit will follow and persevere. To improve as a partner, attempt these tips.

LOVE YOURSELF FIRST

Have you heard the saying "like attracts like"? This is the law of attraction - the idea that we draw in the things that we focus on and encircle ourselves with - and it applies to relationships and life. If you embrace positive reasoning, live with energy, and are caring and tolerate yourself as well as other people, you'll draw in individuals who do likewise. Learning self-love is not simple all the time. You will have to recognize and defeat your limiting convictions and modify your story to invigorate you and give you confidence. Yet, if you are considering how to have a healthy relationship, it's an imperative initial step.

INCREASE YOUR STANDARDS

You must hold yourself to high standards if you need a healthy relationship. If your expectations are low and you're not investing the energy to develop with your partner, the outcome will be an old and crumbling relationship. What do you genuinely need from your relationship? What are the guidelines you'd hold for your fantasy partner? What do you anticipate from your partner, genuinely and inwardly? Anything it is, that is the bar that you should hold for yourself also. You are a functioning member of this relationship; how you believe that they should appear for you is how you should appear for them.

MEET YOUR PARTNER'S CORE NEEDS

What is a healthy relationship? It's two individuals making each other's requirements their own. The more you do this, the seriously satisfying the relationship becomes. What are your partner's center necessities? Solace? Security? Importance? How would they need these requirements met? Through touch, words, or something different? Develop the expertise of ardent comprehension. Going past understanding what your partner needs at a scholarly level, implies interfacing at a more profound emotional level and sympathetically remaining from their point of view. Is your partner your main need? What might you give for your first love? Simultaneously, would you say you are feeling and being satisfied with the relationship?

COMMUNICATE EFFECTIVELY

Healthy relationships rely upon compelling communication. You needn't bother with being telepathic to understand everything that your partner needs - chances are they have said to you. Communicating in a healthy relationship implies listening. Keep in mind, that there's no need to focus on you - it's about how you can help the individual you love. When you understand what your needs are, and your partner's, you can effectively attempt to ensure those needs are being met. How might you help the love of your life? Anything, isn't that so? Meeting your better half's core needs will take you to significant degrees of joy, love, energy, and trust.

DEVELOP TOGETHER

What if the road ahead is tough and brimming with difficulties. As Smith says, "Each problem is a gift, without problems we will not grow." Problems, snags, and misalignments are chances to push forward and develop along with your partner. The absence of development is otherwise called stagnation, which can prompt the crumbling of a relationship. Development is a result of vulnerability and a demonstration of driving into an unfamiliar area. In some cases uneasiness is something to be thankful for, so don't allow dread to hold your relationship - or you - back.

VALUE YOUR DIFFERENCES

You don't have to disregard or make light of the distinctions between you and your partner. Running against the norm, and appreciating your disparities is fundamental to keeping a feeling of energy in the relationship. Those little distinctions stirred your advantage in one another in any case, and this is the sort of thing that you should continuously hold near your souls and psyches. Value one another and you won't just see the value in the existence you have made together - you'll delight in it.

FOSTER TRUST

Trust is the groundwork of all useful and healthy relationships. From trust springs regard, and both are essential for sharing, collaboration, and development. What's more, it's during seasons of pressure and vulnerability, when your common responsibility can be likely uncertainty, that you find how much - or how little - you trust each other.

Might your partner at any point trust you to show up for them, in any event, when you're focused on or unsure? Could your partner at any point trust you to tell the truth and be clear with them, in any event, when you feel like what you need to say could wound them? Do they believe that you will address their issues?

BE HONEST

While contemplating how to have a healthy relationship, honesty is vital - incorporating being straightforward with yourself. Being true to (and confident in) yourself is an essential component in forward-looking conflict resolution in your relationship. It's vital, to tell the truth, and be bold when you face frustration, agony, and shock. The most energetic romances have snapshots of bitterness. Try not to keep away from clashes when they come. Face them genuinely and valiantly, realizing that you and your partner depend on any test.

RETHINK INTIMACY

Intimacy isn't simply physical, and it isn't around 100% of the time "big moments." Real intimacy is about the more modest regular minutes. It's sitting close to each other on the sofa watching your #1 film for the 10th time. It's making your partner's number one feast without them asking you to. Assuming that you end up striving in your endeavors to associate, continue to push. Finding how to keep a healthy relationship implies keeping the flash alive - yet it takes work. Figure out how to convey your contemplations and feelings at the time so you can resolve these issues and try not to seed hatred that will in any case arise later in the relationship.

DISCOVER THE POWER OF POLARITY

Polarity is the attraction between inverse energies. Manly energy is about responsibility, sureness, and reason, though ladylike energy is related to weakness, immediacy, and provocative play. Healthy relationships, regardless of the physical sexes of the partners, need to cooperate with manly energy and ladylike energy. To accomplish enduring enthusiasm with your partner, you need to explore your polarity. It was this polarity that pulled you to one another, and this powerful interplay can keep up passion between you.

ALIGN YOUR VALUES

Indeed, healthy relationships can experience conflicts about values and long-term objectives. A successful relationship will utilize these tough spots as an opportunity to re-adjust and develop, rather than using the conflicts to destroy the relationship.

What are your qualities and objectives, or results? Are the communication patterns and objectives of your partner compatible with yours? Misalignments here can produce friction, yet they are likewise potential chances to develop the relationship to another degree of enthusiasm, intimacy, and association.

SHIFT YOUR FOCUS

If you intend to venture to every part of the turning, deterrent-ridden street toward a healthy relationship, you should be clear to yourself about the result you need; once you accomplish clarity and commitment, you have focus. Where focus goes, energy flows. Will you center around the negatives, or will you put your energy towards solutions? Decide to zero in on solutions, and you will be able to work through problems and celebrate the manner in which your disparities improve your coexistence. You'll start seeing your disparities not as an issue or cause of torment, but rather as a wellspring of joy and energy.

KEEP IT GOING

You've dealt with how to have a healthy relationship and arrived at a fulfilled spot. Now push ahead, showing others how it is done and continuously supporting a healthy, cherishing relationship. You generally have options, regardless of what life tosses your direction. You can encounter agony and endure and rebuff yourself and cooperate with it, or you can take what comes, process it, gain from the experience and sort out some way to apply that illustration to your life. So what is a healthy relationship? Basically, a healthy relationship is something you should support and keep up with, regardless of how long you and your partner are together. Recollect what Smith says: "If you are not developing, you are dying." Experiment, add variety and make a healthy relationship loaded with energy and enthusiasm - and make sure to have a good time!

CHAPTER 6:

MAINTAINING A HEALTHY HOME

It is important that the places we call home are healthy environments, for us as well as our guests. Dangers to health can happen in any home through ecological elements from nature itself, items we use, the air we inhale, or once in a while the food we eat, or the water we drink. An overall counsel to lessen openness to different hurtful substances include:

- Wash your hands with soap and warm water for somewhere around 20 seconds.
- Take off outdoor shoes while entering your home, and request that guests do likewise.
- Decrease residue and soil by vacuuming, cleaning, and wet-wiping consistently.
- Safeguard Visiting Children: Children come into close contact with their

actual environment - creeping on floors, contacting and tasting things. Dust and dirt are key sources of contact with substances like lead, which can influence kids' development even at low degrees of exposure. Make a special effort to have a clean play region for visiting children. Regulate them at all times. It very well may be astonishing what youngsters can be wounded by. Safe handling of medications is important: Keep meds in original containers in secure, cool, dry areas, far away from kids. Continuously use medicine as supervised by your physician or pharmacist. Return extra or terminated prescriptions to your drug store - don't discard them in the sink or latrine.

Home Chemicals

You presumably utilize numerous synthetic items in and around your home, like cleaning items, paints, stains, or windshield washer liquid. Mothballs and moth flakes are stilk being utilized. These items can be hurtful. Read the labels. Search for those warning symbols that indicate that the item could be "perilous". Cautiously follow all security data and headings. Open a close-by window to guarantee satisfactory ventilation while utilizing items like paints, stains, paint strippers, or cleaning items. Take outside air breaks during painting or household renovations.

Mothballs and moth flakes can be hurtful on the off chance that label directions are not followed. Make sure to painstakingly read and follow the package directions. Consider picking low-emission paints, varnishes, and glues. Check with manufacturers for details on specific items. Wear protective gloves to stay away from contact with skin. Purchase just what you want for the task to limit squander. Store chemical items in their unique holders and in protected, secure areas - kept up and out of the reach of children. Discard household hazardous waste products properly. Check with your region about how and where.

Indoor Air Quality

Poor indoor air quality can influence your well-being. Open windows and doors when climate and open-air quality permits to freshen up your home. Maintain your heater and ventilation system by having them examined consistently by a certified technician. Change or clean filters as suggested.

Lessen the Risk of Mould

Mould and damp conditions might irritate your eyes, nose, and throat, and cause coughing, wheezing, and gasping for air. Search for damp spots in your home. Remove small quantities of mould with heated water and dish cleanser. Employ an expert for bigger spaces - the size of half a door, or greater. Keep mould from developing or returning. Fix water leaks and tidy up rapidly after any flood. Ensure everything is dry again in 48 hours or less. Use exhaust fans while cooking and showering.

Ensure your garments dryer, oven, kitchen, and washroom fans all vent to the outside. Eliminate cellar mess. Try not to store texture, food, paper, or wood in sodden regions like a cellar. Utilize plastic capacity containers whenever required. Keep stickiness low - around half in summer and 30% in a colder climate. Utilize a dehumidifier if necessary. Do you lease? Address your landowner about any shape issues. Learn about property manager/inhabitant issues from your commonplace/regional government.

Stay away from Smoke

Smoke harms everybody. The synthetic compounds it contains contribute directly to ailments like asthma, malignant growth, and heart illness. No amount of ventilation will take out the unsafe impacts of smoke. Stay away from openness to recycled tobacco smoke - make your home and vehicle 100 percent smoke-free. Stay away from openness to wood smoke. Wood smoke might smell decent, yet entirely it's not great for you.

Keep Carbon Monoxide Out

Carbon monoxide is a toxic gas that has no variety, smell, or taste. health chances are more prominent for individuals with cardiovascular (or coronary illness. Very elevated degrees of carbon monoxide could prompt demise. Introduce a carbon monoxide caution confirmed by a confirmation body that is certified. Introduce the alert external rooms. Follow the producer's ideas on the most proficient method to introduce, test, use and supplant the caution. Have heaters, chimneys, gas ovens, fireplaces, and water radiators kept up with and reviewed routinely by a prepared proficient. Never utilize a grill inside. Try not to utilize lamp fuel or oil space radiators or lights in encased regions except if they're intended for indoor use. Try not to sit vehicles or different internal combustion machines (e.g., lawnmowers, snowblowers) in the carport, regardless of whether the carport entryway is open.

Beware of Radon

Radon is a gas that can be found in practically all homes. If an individual is exposed to high levels over some years, it can cause lung cancer. Test for it - it's the best way to know the degree of radon gas in your home. You can either buy a long-term, simple-to-utilize radon test pack from a home improvement store, by telephone, or over the Internet, or recruit a certified estimation professional. Fix it assuming that the levels are high. Enlist a certified radon expert to decide the best and most practical method for lessening the radon level in your home.

Safe Food Handling

As we age, our immune system turns out to be less effective and our chances of serious health issues from foodborne and waterborne ailments can increase. Wash your hands before getting food ready. On the off chance that plates or utensils have come into contact with crude food, wash them completely before re-utilizing or use a clean plate. Wash fresh fruits and vegetables with clean drinking water. Wash re-usable staple packs often with hot foamy water, particularly if they've been utilized for raw meat, poultry, fish, or fish. Commit re-usable packs for various purposes - one for meat, poultry, fish, and fish, one for produce, and one for prepared-to-eat food varieties. Name the sacks appropriately.

Clean your refrigerator frequently. Keep it chilled. When you return home from shopping, refrigerate or freeze crude meat, poultry, fish, and fish. Refrigerate extras at the earliest opportunity or in no less than 2 hours in the wake of putting them on the table or counter. Keep store meats refrigerated consistently and use somewhere around 4 days after opening the bundle, regardless of whether this is sooner than the best-before date. Store foods are grown from the ground in the refrigerator. Thaw out your crude meat, poultry, fish, or fish in the ice chest, in the microwave, or chilly water. On the off chance that you've thawed out in the microwave, food ought to be cooked at the earliest opportunity in the wake of defrosting.

While thawing out a huge piece of meat that doesn't fit in the cooler, drench it in chilly water in its unique unopened wrapping. Invigorate the water frequently (for instance, like clockwork) so it stays cold. Don't refreeze defrosted food. Promptly wash hands, sinks, kitchen surfaces, or compartments that interact with crude meat, poultry, fish, or fish. Cook, it completely Uses a computerized food thermometer to guarantee you cook meat, poultry, fish, and fish to a safe interior temperature. Ensure the thermometer goes through the thickest piece of the meat, the whole way to the center, without contacting any bones.

Drinking Water

If you get your drinking water from a well or other sources on your property, ensure it is safe to drink. Water in its natural state generally requires treatment. Drinking bottled water is by and large a safe decision, when handled and stored appropriately. Your district might issue warnings, (for example, "boil water" warnings) when there is a drinking water quality concern. It is critical to painstakingly adhere to guidelines. Contact your district with questions in regards to the treatment or nature of your drinking water. On the off chance that you utilize a pitcher-type water channel, store it in the refrigerator and supplant the channel consistently, as shown in the maker's guidelines.

Has well water been tried by your neighborhood general health division to affirm that it's protected, or what sort of treatment it might require? Buy just treatment gadgets that will address your particular water quality issue; gadgets ought to be affirmed to eliminate explicit foreign substances.

Important: If you use a water conditioner, the softened water ought not to be utilized for drinking or food preparation. It can contain elevated degrees of sodium or potassium - a worry for specific ailments or with certain meds.

Bottled water: Store bottled water in a cool, clean, dim spot, like a storm cellar. Refrigerate the jug after opening to decrease the development of microbes. Store bottled water away from family solvents like acetones or cleaners. Over the long haul, solvents can get high up and go through the plastic jug into the water. Try not to top off water bottles - many were intended for one-time use. Save money on recycling by utilizing a reusable water holder.

Outrageous Heat

On the off chance that it gets excessively hot inside your home, it very well may be hazardous for your health, particularly assuming that you have existing ailments like breathing challenges, heart or kidney issues, hypertension, or experience the ill effects of a mental sickness like depression. Heat stroke is a health-related emergency. Yet, there's uplifting news - heat illnesses are preventable. Know your dangers - consult a doctor or drug specialist to figure out your risk factors and follow their suggestions. Find out about the side effects of heat sickness.

Get ready for heat. Check nearby weather forecasts for heat alarms. Assuming you have a climate control system (or airconditioner), ensure it works before the sweltering weather conditions begin.

Orchestrate visits by relatives or companions during extremely hot days, because you might need help. Remain hydrated. Drink a lot of cool fluids before you feel parched - water is ideal. Eat more leafy foods - they have high water content.

Keep your home cool. On the off chance that you have a forced air system with an indoor regulator, set it somewhere in the range of 22°C and 26°C (72°F and 79°F). On the off chance that you utilize a window climate control system, cool just a single room where you can go for help. Get ready for feasts that don't require cooking on the stove. Block the sun with shades, draperies, or blinds. If protected, open your windows around evening time to allow in cooler air. Remain cool. Wear baggy, light-hued clothing produced using breathable texture.

Consumer Products

Consistently, you use consumer items like personal care items, electronics, clothing, equipment, and cleaning items. Some items can present health risks, so it is critical to focus on warnings, alerts, and recall notices. Know about item recalls - check with the manufacturer. Manage visiting youngsters - ensure you have a protected, clean region where children can play; kids are frequently ignorant about things that can hurt them.

Think security - read marks and adhere to all directions. Try not to utilize harmed, reviewed, or restricted things. Be cautious while purchasing or getting recycled items, including kids' toys. Ensure you get guidelines for use and watch for broken or lacking pieces. Report health or security-related issues with purchased items to the producer.

www.ingramcontent.com/pod-product-compliance
Lightning Source LLC
LaVergne TN
LVHW052047160826
845678LV00015B/3127

* 9 7 9 8 8 4 7 1 0 6 9 0 0 *